THE ULTIMATE MEAL PLANNER

52 Week Food Planner, Journal & Tracker

Published by Encouraging Pen Publications in 2020
First Edition, First Printing
Book Design and Layout © 2020 Jenai Gatlin
Pink Dutch Oven Image from Chimene Gaspar via Pixabay
www.startwithwhatyouvegot.com

ISBN-13: 978-0-9985838-1-5

INDEX

OUR YEAR IN FOOD

Family Name

____

Year

____

COOKING AND MEAL PLANNING STRATEGIES

A recent survey showed that the average American household throws out about $1200 in food per year. Wow! That is really something to think about. Whatever your thoughts on the real problem here, we can all do better in our own households.

The keyword here is "planning." When planning your meals, think of your family's lifestyle and their food preferences. If you are out late or need to eat meals on the go, you will need to prepare differently than someone who has a little longer to spend in the kitchen. You want to be sure not to squander your money on fast foods or lots of expensive convenience foods.

Pantry Staples

I work on the premise that as much as I like to cook, I do not always want to spend a great amount of time in the kitchen. I try to set myself up for success in making home cooked meals (and saving money) by having certain basics on hand. From these basics, I am able to start a meal from scratch or make a meal of what many would consider nothing. I can find a creative use for leftovers or prepare a meal that takes less than 15 minutes and tastes like it took much more time and thought.

To make sure that you have the ingredients on hand that you need to make meals quickly, make a list of the meals that you make most often. Next list the ingredients you need to make those meals. Add the items to your pantry list.

Planned Leftovers

Once I've stocked my pantry, I want to look at the proteins that I've purchased on sale and think about all the ways that I can use them. My other thoughts turn toward keeping my time in the kitchen to a minimum and making sure that I don't throw away the chicken that may be leftover from Sunday's dinner. I don't really want to see the same exact meal three times in one week so I make a plan in advance as to how I will be able to repurpose my food.

For instance, let's say that I have a whole roasted chicken on Sunday. I'll take the rest of the meat from the chicken before putting it away. Tuesday we may have a chicken and spinach lasagna baked in a light cream sauce. On Thursday I'll make a Thai chicken curry or white chicken chili (chicken and white beans). I like to take at least one meal per week and stretch it using this concept.

A pot roast with potatoes, carrots and onions may turn into beef stroganoff, beef enchiladas and beef vegetable soup. A pork loin will be turned into Mu Shu Pork or Lo Mein and BBQ pulled pork sandwiches.

Side dishes can also reappear. Rice will be used later for jambalaya and fried rice. Mashed potatoes can top Shepherd's Pie, be used for potato pancakes, and be used to thicken a soup. Day-old bread becomes a grilled cheese or Panini sandwich, French Toast, bread pudding or a thickener for soup.

The nice thing about all of these new dishes is that there is no real cooking going on. In general, you want to choose dishes that at most call for combining foods that just need to be heated through. For more ideas, do an internet search on "planned leftovers for ______" and see what suggestions you get.

Helpful Tip: To keep food from getting "lost" in your refrigerator, store items in see-though containers so that you can take a quick inventory of what you have and be reminded to use it.

Slow Cookers and Instant Cookers

Pull out that slow or instant cooker that you received as a gift or found on sale. Crockery cooking allows you to use less expensive cuts of meat with fantastic results and gives you the luxury to come home to a home-cooked meal or get one on the table very quickly. Find a specialty cookbook for recipes that will keep you satisfied.

Clean Out the Refrigerator Meals

There are times that you will find yourself with a bunch of hodgepodge items in the refrigerator and you've let your pantry staples get low. For those days, I can still make a meal that doesn't feel like leftovers. I actually make items that we would get in a takeout situation. My arsenal includes:

Burritos – Mix rice, beans, vegetables, meat, cheese with salsa. Put in the center of a flour tortilla, roll and bake. Pour salsa on top. Top with sour cream or guacamole, lettuce and diced tomato.

House Fried Rice or Lo Mein– Rice (or noodles), diced pork, chicken, shrimp and shredded beef stir fried with onions, frozen carrots & peas, soy sauce and eggs.

Pot Pie – Chicken or beef, mixed vegetables, cubed potatoes heated in a white, chicken or beef gravy. Place in a greased casserole dish and top with refrigerated biscuits, raw mixed cornbread or a pie shell crust. Bake until the top crust is done.

"Bowls" – Pick a themed cuisine (Mexican, Mediterranean, Asian, etc.). Start with a base of grains or starch, add a protein, raw greens (like spinach, lettuce, kale), a healthy fat (avocado, hummus, seeds) and other complementary vegetable mix-ins (cooked or raw). Spice it up with herbs, spices and seasonings (like cilantro, basil, lime juice, garlic, hot sauce). Top and stir with a condiments or sauce from your chosen theme (like salsa, tahini, hoisin). You can present the items as a buffet and let each person build their own bowl. This is a perfect way to satisfy picky eaters or a household that has multiple dietary lifestyles.

Choose A Nightly Theme

Try assigning a theme to each night of the week and make a list of meals that fit into that theme (page 116). Your family will have a general idea of what they can expect each night. Themes can be based on world cuisines (Italian, Asian), types of cooking (slow cooker, grilling), and categories of food (pizza, casserole, salad). Try a Meatless Monday, Taco Tuesday, or Breakfast for Dinner night.

Frozen Assets

My husband calls me the Freezer Queen. He jokes that if he stands still too long, he might find himself frozen. I do in fact freeze just about everything. I have meats, all types of berries, bread, herbs, vegetables, and fully cooked meals in my freezer. Freezing works for me because it allows me to buy lots of an item when it is on sale and use it as needed.

I also use the freezer to store items that can be reused in another way later and to freeze leftovers. When I make a meal, I assess how much I think that we will realistically eat over the next few days. If I've made a pot of spaghetti sauce or chili, I know that it is time to pull out the quart sized freezer bags as soon as the pot has cooled. I pack my leftovers in quart sized bags because that is all that we will eat before we tire of it.

Take a few moments each week to plan your meals. Meal planning will help you reduce stress, save you time and save you money. Plus, by taking the time to think about your schedule and meals, you may be able to lose weight and address other health issues that can be controlled with food. Happy Planning!

HOW TO USE THIS BOOK

Each week take a quick inventory of your refrigerator and pantry. This will be your starting point for planning your meals for the week. It will also help you save money by using up what you have first and preventing you from buying duplicate items.

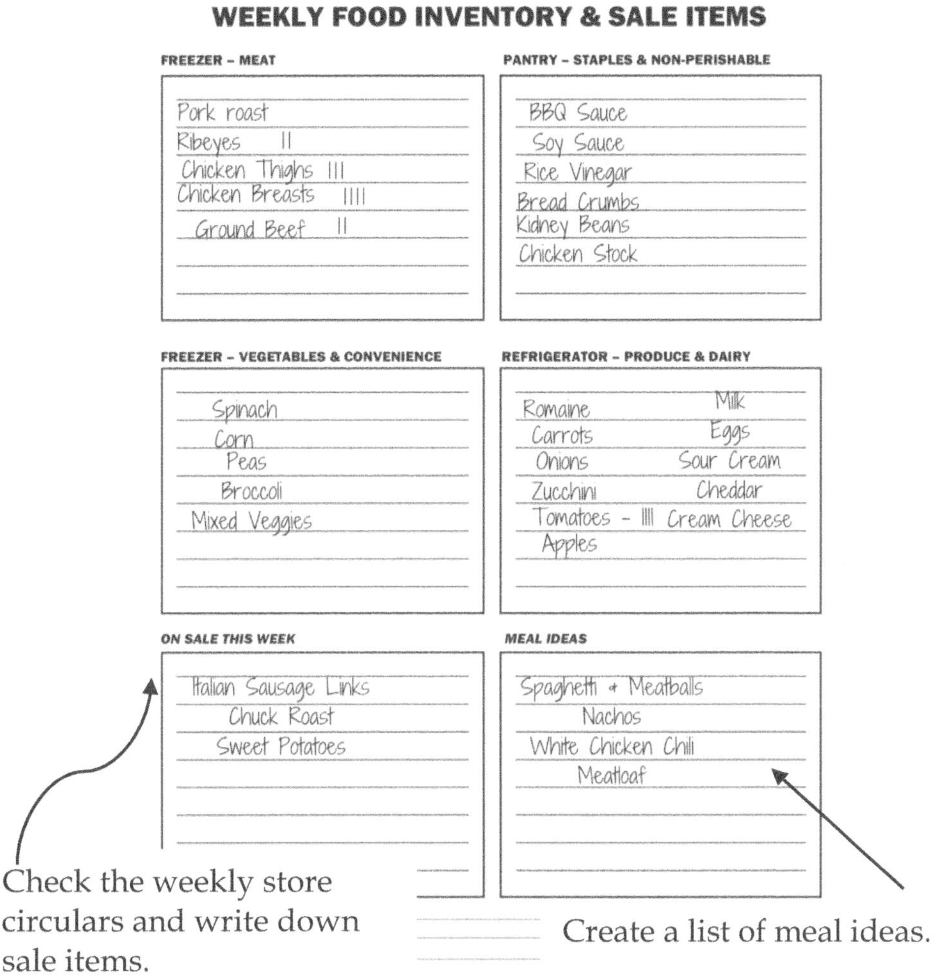
WEEKLY FOOD INVENTORY & SALE ITEMS

FREEZER – MEAT

Pork roast
Ribeyes ||
Chicken Thighs |||
Chicken Breasts ||||
Ground Beef ||

PANTRY – STAPLES & NON-PERISHABLE

BBQ Sauce
Soy Sauce
Rice Vinegar
Bread Crumbs
Kidney Beans
Chicken Stock

FREEZER – VEGETABLES & CONVENIENCE

Spinach
Corn
Peas
Broccoli
Mixed Veggies

REFRIGERATOR – PRODUCE & DAIRY

Romaine — Milk
Carrots — Eggs
Onions — Sour Cream
Zucchini — Cheddar
Tomatoes – |||| — Cream Cheese
Apples

ON SALE THIS WEEK

Italian Sausage Links
Chuck Roast
Sweet Potatoes

MEAL IDEAS

Spaghetti + Meatballs
Nachos
White Chicken Chili
Meatloaf

Next, create your meal plan for the week. Using the inventory on the pages on the left side and the reference sheets starting on page 114, build your menus.

Make note of days that may require special meals such as on the go meals or even scheduling leftovers or breaks from cooking.

You can also keep track of your weekly spending as well as individual prices for specific items. Over time you will notice trends like how often specific items go on sale.

MEAL PLANNER for week of ____________

Budget: $175 Actual: $163 Diff: +$12

Prep/Notes: Sun - Roast 2 chickens, Prep overnight oatmeal for the week Jordyn - Soccer Tues

	BREAKFAST	LUNCH	DINNER	SNACKS
SUN	Brunch- Monte Cristo Sandwiches		Roast Chicken Green Beans Mashed Potatoes	
MON	Overnight Oats Raspberries	Chicken Caesar Wraps	Chicken Cutlets Sweet Potatoes Broccoli	Boiled Eggs
TUE	Boiled Eggs Toast	Chicken Salad Sandwich Grapes	TACO TUESDAY Slow Cooker Chix Fajitas Tortillas, Zucchini	Cheese Crackers
WED	Overnight Oats Blueberries	Buffalo Chicken Strips Oven Baked Fries	Spaghetti + Meatballs Salad	
THU	Fruit Smoothies	Chicken Salad Sandwich Carrots	LEFTOVER MAKEOVER Fried Rice with leftover meats and veggies	Tortilla Chips Salsa
FRI	Overnight Oats Bananas	BBQ Chicken Sandwich Chips	Takeout - Chinese	
SAT	Waffles Bacon	ON YOUR OWN!	Pizza Salad	

Be sure to take time to record your favorites and go-to meals. The more you use this book, the easier planning will be.

You may find it easier to use this book with spiral binding. Simply take this planner to your local office supply store or copy shop and have them bind it for you.

FREE GIFT!

As a thank you for purchasing this planner, I have a **free gift for you**. Download free stickers to complement your menu planning at www.startwithwhatyouvegot.com.

PANTRY STAPLES

PRODUCE (FRESH)

Apples
Avocados
Bananas
Carrots
Celery
Cilantro
Lemons
Leafy Greens
Lettuce
Garlic
Onions
Potatoes
Tomatoes

FREEZER

Berries
Broccoli
Corn
Peas
Spinach
Juice
Puff Pastry
Vanilla Ice Cream

CANNED GOODS

Chicken Broth/Stock
Beans
Corn
Olives
Chiles or Pickled Jalapenos
Salsa
Tomatoes & Sauce
Tuna

DAIRY

Butter, Unsalted
Cheese - Cheddar, Mozz
Parmesan Cheese
Milk
Eggs
Sour Cream
Yogurt

MEAT

Ground Meat
Chicken
Bacon

GRAINS

Long Grain White Rice
Brown Rice
Grain - Quinoa, Couscous
Pasta
Oats
Polenta or Grits
Breadcrumbs
Dried Beans
Bread

CONDIMENTS

Hot Sauce
Jelly/Jam
Honey
Maple Syrup
Ketchup
Mustard
Mayonnaise
Nut Butters
Pickles
Soy Sauce
Worcestershire Sauce

SNACKS

Breakfast Cereal
Cookies
Crackers
Dried Fruit
Nuts
Popcorn
Tortillas
Tortilla Chips

BAKING GOODS

Flour
Baking Soda
Baking Powder
Cocoa Powder (unsweetened)
Chocolate
Evaporated Milk
Vanilla Extract
Brown Sugar
Granulated Sugar
Confectioners' Sugar

OILS/VINEGARS

Olive Oil
Vegetable Oil
Coconut Oil
Apple Cider Vinegar
Balsamic Vinegar
Red Wine Vinegar
Rice Wine Vinegar
White Vinegar

HERBS & SPICES

Bay Leaves
Basil
Black Pepper
Cayenne
Cinnamon
Chili Powder
Cumin
Garlic Powder
Ginger (Ground)
Nutmeg
Onion Powder
Oregano
Paprika
Salt
Thyme

WEEKLY FOOD INVENTORY & SALE ITEMS

FREEZER – MEAT

PANTRY – STAPLES & NON-PERISHABLE

FREEZER – VEGETABLES & CONVENIENCE

REFRIGERATOR – PRODUCE & DAIRY

ON SALE THIS WEEK

MEAL IDEAS

MEAL PLANNER for week of ____________________

Budget: ________________ Actual: ________________ Diff: ____________

Prep/Notes: ____

____

	BREAKFAST	LUNCH	DINNER	SNACKS
SUN				
MON				
TUE				
WED				
THU				
FRI				
SAT				

WEEKLY FOOD INVENTORY & SALE ITEMS

FREEZER – MEAT

PANTRY – STAPLES & NON-PERISHABLE

FREEZER – VEGETABLES & CONVENIENCE

REFRIGERATOR – PRODUCE & DAIRY

ON SALE THIS WEEK

MEAL IDEAS

MEAL PLANNER for week of ______________________

Budget: _______________ Actual: _______________ Diff: ___________

Prep/Notes: ____

____

	BREAKFAST	LUNCH	DINNER	SNACKS
SUN				
MON				
TUE				
WED				
THU				
FRI				
SAT				

WEEKLY FOOD INVENTORY & SALE ITEMS

FREEZER – MEAT

PANTRY – STAPLES & NON-PERISHABLE

FREEZER – VEGETABLES & CONVENIENCE

REFRIGERATOR – PRODUCE & DAIRY

ON SALE THIS WEEK

MEAL IDEAS

MEAL PLANNER for week of ______________________

Budget: ________________ Actual: ________________ Diff: ____________

Prep/Notes: ____

____

	BREAKFAST	LUNCH	DINNER	SNACKS
SUN				
MON				
TUE				
WED				
THU				
FRI				
SAT				

WEEKLY FOOD INVENTORY & SALE ITEMS

FREEZER – MEAT

PANTRY – STAPLES & NON-PERISHABLE

FREEZER – VEGETABLES & CONVENIENCE

REFRIGERATOR – PRODUCE & DAIRY

ON SALE THIS WEEK

MEAL IDEAS

MEAL PLANNER for week of ______________________

Budget: ______________ Actual: ______________ Diff: __________

Prep/Notes: ____

____

	BREAKFAST	LUNCH	DINNER	SNACKS
SUN				
MON				
TUE				
WED				
THU				
FRI				
SAT				

WEEKLY FOOD INVENTORY & SALE ITEMS

FREEZER – MEAT

PANTRY – STAPLES & NON-PERISHABLE

FREEZER – VEGETABLES & CONVENIENCE

REFRIGERATOR – PRODUCE & DAIRY

ON SALE THIS WEEK

MEAL IDEAS

MEAL PLANNER for week of ____________________

Budget: ______________ Actual: ______________ Diff: __________

Prep/Notes: ____

____

	BREAKFAST	LUNCH	DINNER	SNACKS
SUN				
MON				
TUE				
WED				
THU				
FRI				
SAT				

WEEKLY FOOD INVENTORY & SALE ITEMS

FREEZER – MEAT

PANTRY – STAPLES & NON-PERISHABLE

FREEZER – VEGETABLES & CONVENIENCE

REFRIGERATOR – PRODUCE & DAIRY

ON SALE THIS WEEK

MEAL IDEAS

MEAL PLANNER for week of ____________________

Budget: ______________ Actual: ______________ Diff: __________

Prep/Notes: ____

____

	BREAKFAST	LUNCH	DINNER	SNACKS
SUN				
MON				
TUE				
WED				
THU				
FRI				
SAT				

WEEKLY FOOD INVENTORY & SALE ITEMS

FREEZER – MEAT

PANTRY – STAPLES & NON-PERISHABLE

FREEZER – VEGETABLES & CONVENIENCE

REFRIGERATOR – PRODUCE & DAIRY

ON SALE THIS WEEK

MEAL IDEAS

MEAL PLANNER for week of ____________________

Budget: ________________ Actual: ________________ Diff: ____________

Prep/Notes: ____

____

	BREAKFAST	LUNCH	DINNER	SNACKS
SUN				
MON				
TUE				
WED				
THU				
FRI				
SAT				

WEEKLY FOOD INVENTORY & SALE ITEMS

FREEZER – MEAT

PANTRY – STAPLES & NON-PERISHABLE

FREEZER – VEGETABLES & CONVENIENCE

REFRIGERATOR – PRODUCE & DAIRY

ON SALE THIS WEEK

MEAL IDEAS

MEAL PLANNER for week of ____________________

Budget: ________________ Actual: ________________ Diff: ____________

Prep/Notes: ____

____

	BREAKFAST	LUNCH	DINNER	SNACKS
SUN				
MON				
TUE				
WED				
THU				
FRI				
SAT				

WEEKLY FOOD INVENTORY & SALE ITEMS

FREEZER – MEAT

PANTRY – STAPLES & NON-PERISHABLE

FREEZER – VEGETABLES & CONVENIENCE

REFRIGERATOR – PRODUCE & DAIRY

ON SALE THIS WEEK

MEAL IDEAS

MEAL PLANNER for week of ____________________

Budget: ________________ Actual: ________________ Diff: ____________

Prep/Notes: ____

____

	BREAKFAST	LUNCH	DINNER	SNACKS
SUN				
MON				
TUE				
WED				
THU				
FRI				
SAT				

WEEKLY FOOD INVENTORY & SALE ITEMS

FREEZER – MEAT

PANTRY – STAPLES & NON-PERISHABLE

FREEZER – VEGETABLES & CONVENIENCE

REFRIGERATOR – PRODUCE & DAIRY

ON SALE THIS WEEK

MEAL IDEAS

MEAL PLANNER for week of ____________________

Budget: _______________ Actual: _______________ Diff: ___________

Prep/Notes: ____

____

	BREAKFAST	LUNCH	DINNER	SNACKS
SUN				
MON				
TUE				
WED				
THU				
FRI				
SAT				

WEEKLY FOOD INVENTORY & SALE ITEMS

FREEZER – MEAT

PANTRY – STAPLES & NON-PERISHABLE

FREEZER – VEGETABLES & CONVENIENCE

REFRIGERATOR – PRODUCE & DAIRY

ON SALE THIS WEEK

MEAL IDEAS

MEAL PLANNER for week of ____________________

Budget: ________________ Actual: ________________ Diff: ____________

Prep/Notes: ____

____

	BREAKFAST	LUNCH	DINNER	SNACKS
SUN				
MON				
TUE				
WED				
THU				
FRI				
SAT				

WEEKLY FOOD INVENTORY & SALE ITEMS

FREEZER – MEAT

PANTRY – STAPLES & NON-PERISHABLE

FREEZER – VEGETABLES & CONVENIENCE

REFRIGERATOR – PRODUCE & DAIRY

ON SALE THIS WEEK

MEAL IDEAS

MEAL PLANNER for week of ____________________

Budget: ______________ Actual: ______________ Diff: __________

Prep/Notes: ____

____

	BREAKFAST	LUNCH	DINNER	SNACKS
SUN				
MON				
TUE				
WED				
THU				
FRI				
SAT				

WEEKLY FOOD INVENTORY & SALE ITEMS

FREEZER – MEAT

PANTRY – STAPLES & NON-PERISHABLE

FREEZER – VEGETABLES & CONVENIENCE

REFRIGERATOR – PRODUCE & DAIRY

ON SALE THIS WEEK

MEAL IDEAS

MEAL PLANNER for week of ____________________

Budget: ________________ Actual: ________________ Diff: ____________

Prep/Notes: ____

____

	BREAKFAST	LUNCH	DINNER	SNACKS
SUN				
MON				
TUE				
WED				
THU				
FRI				
SAT				

WEEKLY FOOD INVENTORY & SALE ITEMS

FREEZER – MEAT

PANTRY – STAPLES & NON-PERISHABLE

FREEZER – VEGETABLES & CONVENIENCE

REFRIGERATOR – PRODUCE & DAIRY

ON SALE THIS WEEK

MEAL IDEAS

MEAL PLANNER for week of ____________________

Budget: ______________ Actual: ______________ Diff: __________

Prep/Notes: ____

____

	BREAKFAST	LUNCH	DINNER	SNACKS
SUN				
MON				
TUE				
WED				
THU				
FRI				
SAT				

WEEKLY FOOD INVENTORY & SALE ITEMS

FREEZER – MEAT

PANTRY – STAPLES & NON-PERISHABLE

FREEZER – VEGETABLES & CONVENIENCE

REFRIGERATOR – PRODUCE & DAIRY

ON SALE THIS WEEK

MEAL IDEAS

MEAL PLANNER for week of ____________________

Budget: ______________ Actual: ______________ Diff: __________

Prep/Notes: ____

____

	BREAKFAST	LUNCH	DINNER	SNACKS
SUN				
MON				
TUE				
WED				
THU				
FRI				
SAT				

WEEKLY FOOD INVENTORY & SALE ITEMS

FREEZER – MEAT

PANTRY – STAPLES & NON-PERISHABLE

FREEZER – VEGETABLES & CONVENIENCE

REFRIGERATOR – PRODUCE & DAIRY

ON SALE THIS WEEK

MEAL IDEAS

MEAL PLANNER for week of ____________________

Budget: ________________ Actual: ________________ Diff: ____________

Prep/Notes: ____

____

	BREAKFAST	LUNCH	DINNER	SNACKS
SUN				
MON				
TUE				
WED				
THU				
FRI				
SAT				

WEEKLY FOOD INVENTORY & SALE ITEMS

FREEZER – MEAT

PANTRY – STAPLES & NON-PERISHABLE

FREEZER – VEGETABLES & CONVENIENCE

REFRIGERATOR – PRODUCE & DAIRY

ON SALE THIS WEEK

MEAL IDEAS

MEAL PLANNER for week of ____________________

Budget: ________________ Actual: ________________ Diff: ____________

Prep/Notes: ____

____

	BREAKFAST	LUNCH	DINNER	SNACKS
SUN				
MON				
TUE				
WED				
THU				
FRI				
SAT				

WEEKLY FOOD INVENTORY & SALE ITEMS

FREEZER – MEAT

PANTRY – STAPLES & NON-PERISHABLE

FREEZER – VEGETABLES & CONVENIENCE

REFRIGERATOR – PRODUCE & DAIRY

ON SALE THIS WEEK

MEAL IDEAS

MEAL PLANNER for week of ____________________

Budget: ________________ Actual: ________________ Diff: ____________

Prep/Notes: ____

____

	BREAKFAST	LUNCH	DINNER	SNACKS
SUN				
MON				
TUE				
WED				
THU				
FRI				
SAT				

WEEKLY FOOD INVENTORY & SALE ITEMS

FREEZER – MEAT

PANTRY – STAPLES & NON-PERISHABLE

FREEZER – VEGETABLES & CONVENIENCE

REFRIGERATOR – PRODUCE & DAIRY

ON SALE THIS WEEK

MEAL IDEAS

MEAL PLANNER for week of ____________________

Budget: ________________ Actual: ________________ Diff: ____________

Prep/Notes: ____

____

	BREAKFAST	LUNCH	DINNER	SNACKS
SUN				
MON				
TUE				
WED				
THU				
FRI				
SAT				

WEEKLY FOOD INVENTORY & SALE ITEMS

FREEZER – MEAT

PANTRY – STAPLES & NON-PERISHABLE

FREEZER – VEGETABLES & CONVENIENCE

REFRIGERATOR – PRODUCE & DAIRY

ON SALE THIS WEEK

MEAL IDEAS

MEAL PLANNER for week of ____________________

Budget: ______________ Actual: ______________ Diff: __________

Prep/Notes: ____

____

	BREAKFAST	LUNCH	DINNER	SNACKS
SUN				
MON				
TUE				
WED				
THU				
FRI				
SAT				

WEEKLY FOOD INVENTORY & SALE ITEMS

FREEZER – MEAT

PANTRY – STAPLES & NON-PERISHABLE

FREEZER – VEGETABLES & CONVENIENCE

REFRIGERATOR – PRODUCE & DAIRY

ON SALE THIS WEEK

MEAL IDEAS

MEAL PLANNER for week of ____________________

Budget: ______________ Actual: ______________ Diff: __________

Prep/Notes: ____

____

	BREAKFAST	LUNCH	DINNER	SNACKS
SUN				
MON				
TUE				
WED				
THU				
FRI				
SAT				

WEEKLY FOOD INVENTORY & SALE ITEMS

FREEZER – MEAT

PANTRY – STAPLES & NON-PERISHABLE

FREEZER – VEGETABLES & CONVENIENCE

REFRIGERATOR – PRODUCE & DAIRY

ON SALE THIS WEEK

MEAL IDEAS

MEAL PLANNER for week of ____________________

Budget: ________________ Actual: ________________ Diff: ____________

Prep/Notes: ____

____

	BREAKFAST	LUNCH	DINNER	SNACKS
SUN				
MON				
TUE				
WED				
THU				
FRI				
SAT				

WEEKLY FOOD INVENTORY & SALE ITEMS

FREEZER – MEAT

PANTRY – STAPLES & NON-PERISHABLE

FREEZER – VEGETABLES & CONVENIENCE

REFRIGERATOR – PRODUCE & DAIRY

ON SALE THIS WEEK

MEAL IDEAS

MEAL PLANNER for week of ____________________

Budget: ________________ Actual: ________________ Diff: ____________

Prep/Notes: ____

____

	BREAKFAST	LUNCH	DINNER	SNACKS
SUN				
MON				
TUE				
WED				
THU				
FRI				
SAT				

WEEKLY FOOD INVENTORY & SALE ITEMS

FREEZER – MEAT

PANTRY – STAPLES & NON-PERISHABLE

FREEZER – VEGETABLES & CONVENIENCE

REFRIGERATOR – PRODUCE & DAIRY

ON SALE THIS WEEK

MEAL IDEAS

MEAL PLANNER for week of ____________________

Budget: ____________________ Actual: ____________________ Diff: ______________

Prep/Notes: ____

____

	BREAKFAST	LUNCH	DINNER	SNACKS
SUN				
MON				
TUE				
WED				
THU				
FRI				
SAT				

WEEKLY FOOD INVENTORY & SALE ITEMS

FREEZER – MEAT

PANTRY – STAPLES & NON-PERISHABLE

FREEZER – VEGETABLES & CONVENIENCE

REFRIGERATOR – PRODUCE & DAIRY

ON SALE THIS WEEK

MEAL IDEAS

MEAL PLANNER for week of ____________________

Budget: ____________ Actual: ____________ Diff: __________

Prep/Notes: ____

____

	BREAKFAST	LUNCH	DINNER	SNACKS
SUN				
MON				
TUE				
WED				
THU				
FRI				
SAT				

WEEKLY FOOD INVENTORY & SALE ITEMS

FREEZER – MEAT

PANTRY – STAPLES & NON-PERISHABLE

FREEZER – VEGETABLES & CONVENIENCE

REFRIGERATOR – PRODUCE & DAIRY

ON SALE THIS WEEK

MEAL IDEAS

MEAL PLANNER for week of ____________________

Budget: ______________ Actual: ______________ Diff: __________

Prep/Notes: ____

____

	BREAKFAST	LUNCH	DINNER	SNACKS
SUN				
MON				
TUE				
WED				
THU				
FRI				
SAT				

WEEKLY FOOD INVENTORY & SALE ITEMS

FREEZER – MEAT

PANTRY – STAPLES & NON-PERISHABLE

FREEZER – VEGETABLES & CONVENIENCE

REFRIGERATOR – PRODUCE & DAIRY

ON SALE THIS WEEK

MEAL IDEAS

MEAL PLANNER for week of ____________________

Budget: ________________ Actual: ________________ Diff: ____________

Prep/Notes: ____

____

	BREAKFAST	LUNCH	DINNER	SNACKS
SUN				
MON				
TUE				
WED				
THU				
FRI				
SAT				

WEEKLY FOOD INVENTORY & SALE ITEMS

FREEZER – MEAT

PANTRY – STAPLES & NON-PERISHABLE

FREEZER – VEGETABLES & CONVENIENCE

REFRIGERATOR – PRODUCE & DAIRY

ON SALE THIS WEEK

MEAL IDEAS

MEAL PLANNER for week of ______________________

Budget: ________________ Actual: ________________ Diff: ____________

Prep/Notes: ____

____

	BREAKFAST	LUNCH	DINNER	SNACKS
SUN				
MON				
TUE				
WED				
THU				
FRI				
SAT				

WEEKLY FOOD INVENTORY & SALE ITEMS

FREEZER – MEAT

PANTRY – STAPLES & NON-PERISHABLE

FREEZER – VEGETABLES & CONVENIENCE

REFRIGERATOR – PRODUCE & DAIRY

ON SALE THIS WEEK

MEAL IDEAS

MEAL PLANNER for week of ____________________

Budget: ________________ Actual: ________________ Diff: ____________

Prep/Notes: ____

____

	BREAKFAST	LUNCH	DINNER	SNACKS
SUN				
MON				
TUE				
WED				
THU				
FRI				
SAT				

WEEKLY FOOD INVENTORY & SALE ITEMS

FREEZER – MEAT

PANTRY – STAPLES & NON-PERISHABLE

FREEZER – VEGETABLES & CONVENIENCE

REFRIGERATOR – PRODUCE & DAIRY

ON SALE THIS WEEK

MEAL IDEAS

MEAL PLANNER for week of ____________________

Budget: ______________ Actual: ______________ Diff: __________

Prep/Notes: ____

____

	BREAKFAST	LUNCH	DINNER	SNACKS
SUN				
MON				
TUE				
WED				
THU				
FRI				
SAT				

WEEKLY FOOD INVENTORY & SALE ITEMS

FREEZER – MEAT

PANTRY – STAPLES & NON-PERISHABLE

FREEZER – VEGETABLES & CONVENIENCE

REFRIGERATOR – PRODUCE & DAIRY

ON SALE THIS WEEK

MEAL IDEAS

MEAL PLANNER for week of ____________________

Budget: ______________ Actual: ______________ Diff: __________

Prep/Notes: ____

____

	BREAKFAST	LUNCH	DINNER	SNACKS
SUN				
MON				
TUE				
WED				
THU				
FRI				
SAT				

WEEKLY FOOD INVENTORY & SALE ITEMS

FREEZER – MEAT

PANTRY – STAPLES & NON-PERISHABLE

FREEZER – VEGETABLES & CONVENIENCE

REFRIGERATOR – PRODUCE & DAIRY

ON SALE THIS WEEK

MEAL IDEAS

MEAL PLANNER for week of ____________________

Budget: ________________ Actual: ________________ Diff: ____________

Prep/Notes: ____

____

	BREAKFAST	LUNCH	DINNER	SNACKS
SUN				
MON				
TUE				
WED				
THU				
FRI				
SAT				

WEEKLY FOOD INVENTORY & SALE ITEMS

FREEZER – MEAT

PANTRY – STAPLES & NON-PERISHABLE

FREEZER – VEGETABLES & CONVENIENCE

REFRIGERATOR – PRODUCE & DAIRY

ON SALE THIS WEEK

MEAL IDEAS

MEAL PLANNER for week of ____________________

Budget: ______________ Actual: ______________ Diff: __________

Prep/Notes: ____

____

	BREAKFAST	LUNCH	DINNER	SNACKS
SUN				
MON				
TUE				
WED				
THU				
FRI				
SAT				

WEEKLY FOOD INVENTORY & SALE ITEMS

FREEZER – MEAT

PANTRY – STAPLES & NON-PERISHABLE

FREEZER – VEGETABLES & CONVENIENCE

REFRIGERATOR – PRODUCE & DAIRY

ON SALE THIS WEEK

MEAL IDEAS

MEAL PLANNER for week of ____________________

Budget: ______________ Actual: ______________ Diff: __________

Prep/Notes: ____

____

	BREAKFAST	LUNCH	DINNER	SNACKS
SUN				
MON				
TUE				
WED				
THU				
FRI				
SAT				

WEEKLY FOOD INVENTORY & SALE ITEMS

FREEZER – MEAT

PANTRY – STAPLES & NON-PERISHABLE

FREEZER – VEGETABLES & CONVENIENCE

REFRIGERATOR – PRODUCE & DAIRY

ON SALE THIS WEEK

MEAL IDEAS

MEAL PLANNER for week of ____________________

Budget: ________________ Actual: ________________ Diff: ____________

Prep/Notes: ____

____

	BREAKFAST	**LUNCH**	**DINNER**	**SNACKS**
SUN				
MON				
TUE				
WED				
THU				
FRI				
SAT				

WEEKLY FOOD INVENTORY & SALE ITEMS

FREEZER – MEAT

PANTRY – STAPLES & NON-PERISHABLE

FREEZER – VEGETABLES & CONVENIENCE

REFRIGERATOR – PRODUCE & DAIRY

ON SALE THIS WEEK

MEAL IDEAS

MEAL PLANNER for week of ____________________

Budget: ________________ Actual: ________________ Diff: ____________

Prep/Notes: ____

____

	BREAKFAST	LUNCH	DINNER	SNACKS
SUN				
MON				
TUE				
WED				
THU				
FRI				
SAT				

WEEKLY FOOD INVENTORY & SALE ITEMS

FREEZER – MEAT

PANTRY – STAPLES & NON-PERISHABLE

FREEZER – VEGETABLES & CONVENIENCE

REFRIGERATOR – PRODUCE & DAIRY

ON SALE THIS WEEK

MEAL IDEAS

MEAL PLANNER for week of ____________________

Budget: ____________________ Actual: ____________________ Diff: ______________

Prep/Notes: ____

____

	BREAKFAST	LUNCH	DINNER	SNACKS
SUN				
MON				
TUE				
WED				
THU				
FRI				
SAT				

WEEKLY FOOD INVENTORY & SALE ITEMS

FREEZER – MEAT

PANTRY – STAPLES & NON-PERISHABLE

FREEZER – VEGETABLES & CONVENIENCE

REFRIGERATOR – PRODUCE & DAIRY

ON SALE THIS WEEK

MEAL IDEAS

MEAL PLANNER for week of ____________________

Budget: ________________ Actual: ________________ Diff: ____________

Prep/Notes: ____

____

	BREAKFAST	LUNCH	DINNER	SNACKS
SUN				
MON				
TUE				
WED				
THU				
FRI				
SAT				

WEEKLY FOOD INVENTORY & SALE ITEMS

FREEZER – MEAT

PANTRY – STAPLES & NON-PERISHABLE

FREEZER – VEGETABLES & CONVENIENCE

REFRIGERATOR – PRODUCE & DAIRY

ON SALE THIS WEEK

MEAL IDEAS

MEAL PLANNER for week of ____________________

Budget: ______________ Actual: ______________ Diff: __________

Prep/Notes: ____

____

	BREAKFAST	LUNCH	DINNER	SNACKS
SUN				
MON				
TUE				
WED				
THU				
FRI				
SAT				

WEEKLY FOOD INVENTORY & SALE ITEMS

FREEZER – MEAT

PANTRY – STAPLES & NON-PERISHABLE

FREEZER – VEGETABLES & CONVENIENCE

REFRIGERATOR – PRODUCE & DAIRY

ON SALE THIS WEEK

MEAL IDEAS

MEAL PLANNER for week of ______________________

Budget: ________________ Actual: ________________ Diff: ____________

Prep/Notes: ____

____

	BREAKFAST	LUNCH	DINNER	SNACKS
SUN				
MON				
TUE				
WED				
THU				
FRI				
SAT				

WEEKLY FOOD INVENTORY & SALE ITEMS

FREEZER – MEAT

PANTRY – STAPLES & NON-PERISHABLE

FREEZER – VEGETABLES & CONVENIENCE

REFRIGERATOR – PRODUCE & DAIRY

ON SALE THIS WEEK

MEAL IDEAS

MEAL PLANNER for week of ____________________

Budget: ______________ Actual: ______________ Diff: __________

Prep/Notes: ____

____

	BREAKFAST	LUNCH	DINNER	SNACKS
SUN				
MON				
TUE				
WED				
THU				
FRI				
SAT				

WEEKLY FOOD INVENTORY & SALE ITEMS

FREEZER – MEAT

PANTRY – STAPLES & NON-PERISHABLE

FREEZER – VEGETABLES & CONVENIENCE

REFRIGERATOR – PRODUCE & DAIRY

ON SALE THIS WEEK

MEAL IDEAS

MEAL PLANNER for week of ____________________

Budget: _______________ Actual: _______________ Diff: ___________

Prep/Notes: ____

____

	BREAKFAST	LUNCH	DINNER	SNACKS
SUN				
MON				
TUE				
WED				
THU				
FRI				
SAT				

WEEKLY FOOD INVENTORY & SALE ITEMS

FREEZER – MEAT

PANTRY – STAPLES & NON-PERISHABLE

FREEZER – VEGETABLES & CONVENIENCE

REFRIGERATOR – PRODUCE & DAIRY

ON SALE THIS WEEK

MEAL IDEAS

MEAL PLANNER for week of ____________________

Budget: ________________ Actual: ________________ Diff: ____________

Prep/Notes: ____

____

	BREAKFAST	LUNCH	DINNER	SNACKS
SUN				
MON				
TUE				
WED				
THU				
FRI				
SAT				

WEEKLY FOOD INVENTORY & SALE ITEMS

FREEZER – MEAT

PANTRY – STAPLES & NON-PERISHABLE

FREEZER – VEGETABLES & CONVENIENCE

REFRIGERATOR – PRODUCE & DAIRY

ON SALE THIS WEEK

MEAL IDEAS

MEAL PLANNER for week of ______________________

Budget: ________________ Actual: ________________ Diff: ____________

Prep/Notes: ____

____

	BREAKFAST	LUNCH	DINNER	SNACKS
SUN				
MON				
TUE				
WED				
THU				
FRI				
SAT				

WEEKLY FOOD INVENTORY & SALE ITEMS

FREEZER – MEAT

PANTRY – STAPLES & NON-PERISHABLE

FREEZER – VEGETABLES & CONVENIENCE

REFRIGERATOR – PRODUCE & DAIRY

ON SALE THIS WEEK

MEAL IDEAS

MEAL PLANNER for week of ____________________

Budget: ________________ Actual: ________________ Diff: ____________

Prep/Notes: ____

____

	BREAKFAST	LUNCH	DINNER	SNACKS
SUN				
MON				
TUE				
WED				
THU				
FRI				
SAT				

WEEKLY FOOD INVENTORY & SALE ITEMS

FREEZER – MEAT

PANTRY – STAPLES & NON-PERISHABLE

FREEZER – VEGETABLES & CONVENIENCE

REFRIGERATOR – PRODUCE & DAIRY

ON SALE THIS WEEK

MEAL IDEAS

MEAL PLANNER for week of ____________________

Budget: ______________ Actual: ______________ Diff: __________

Prep/Notes: ____

____

	BREAKFAST	LUNCH	DINNER	SNACKS
SUN				
MON				
TUE				
WED				
THU				
FRI				
SAT				

WEEKLY FOOD INVENTORY & SALE ITEMS

FREEZER – MEAT

PANTRY – STAPLES & NON-PERISHABLE

FREEZER – VEGETABLES & CONVENIENCE

REFRIGERATOR – PRODUCE & DAIRY

ON SALE THIS WEEK

MEAL IDEAS

MEAL PLANNER for week of ____________________

Budget: ______________ Actual: ______________ Diff: ____________

Prep/Notes: ____

____

	BREAKFAST	LUNCH	DINNER	SNACKS
SUN				
MON				
TUE				
WED				
THU				
FRI				
SAT				

WEEKLY FOOD INVENTORY & SALE ITEMS

FREEZER – MEAT

PANTRY – STAPLES & NON-PERISHABLE

FREEZER – VEGETABLES & CONVENIENCE

REFRIGERATOR – PRODUCE & DAIRY

ON SALE THIS WEEK

MEAL IDEAS

MEAL PLANNER for week of ____________________

Budget: ________________ Actual: ________________ Diff: ____________

Prep/Notes: ____

____

	BREAKFAST	LUNCH	DINNER	SNACKS
SUN				
MON				
TUE				
WED				
THU				
FRI				
SAT				

WEEKLY FOOD INVENTORY & SALE ITEMS

FREEZER – MEAT

PANTRY – STAPLES & NON-PERISHABLE

FREEZER – VEGETABLES & CONVENIENCE

REFRIGERATOR – PRODUCE & DAIRY

ON SALE THIS WEEK

MEAL IDEAS

MEAL PLANNER for week of ____________________

Budget: ________________ Actual: ________________ Diff: ____________

Prep/Notes: ____

____

	BREAKFAST	LUNCH	DINNER	SNACKS
SUN				
MON				
TUE				
WED				
THU				
FRI				
SAT				

WEEKLY FOOD INVENTORY & SALE ITEMS

FREEZER – MEAT

PANTRY – STAPLES & NON-PERISHABLE

FREEZER – VEGETABLES & CONVENIENCE

REFRIGERATOR – PRODUCE & DAIRY

ON SALE THIS WEEK

MEAL IDEAS

MEAL PLANNER for week of ____________________

Budget: ________________ Actual: ________________ Diff: ____________

Prep/Notes: ____

____

	BREAKFAST	LUNCH	DINNER	SNACKS
SUN				
MON				
TUE				
WED				
THU				
FRI				
SAT				

WEEKLY FOOD INVENTORY & SALE ITEMS

FREEZER – MEAT

PANTRY – STAPLES & NON-PERISHABLE

FREEZER – VEGETABLES & CONVENIENCE

REFRIGERATOR – PRODUCE & DAIRY

ON SALE THIS WEEK

MEAL IDEAS

MEAL PLANNER for week of ____________________

Budget: ____________________ Actual: ____________________ Diff: ______________

Prep/Notes: ____

____

	BREAKFAST	LUNCH	DINNER	SNACKS
SUN				
MON				
TUE				
WED				
THU				
FRI				
SAT				

WEEKLY FOOD INVENTORY & SALE ITEMS

FREEZER – MEAT

PANTRY – STAPLES & NON-PERISHABLE

FREEZER – VEGETABLES & CONVENIENCE

REFRIGERATOR – PRODUCE & DAIRY

ON SALE THIS WEEK

MEAL IDEAS

MEAL PLANNER for week of ____________________

Budget: ______________ Actual: ______________ Diff: __________

Prep/Notes: ____

____

	BREAKFAST	LUNCH	DINNER	SNACKS
SUN				
MON				
TUE				
WED				
THU				
FRI				
SAT				

OUR FAVORITE MEALS

	BREAKFAST	LUNCH	DINNER
NAME			
NAME			
NAME			
NAME			
NAME			

MEAL IDEAS

GROUND MEAT

CHICKEN

SIDE DISHES

SLOW COOKER

CASSEROLES

ON-THE-GO

THEMED MEAL IDEAS

MEATLESS MONDAY

TACO TUESDAY

OUR GO-TO MEALS

BREAKFAST

LUNCH

DINNER

DESSERTS

SNACKS

UNDER 30 MINUTES

RESTAURANT TAKE-OUT MEALS

RESTAURANT	PHONE #	FAVORITE DISHES

MEALS FOR WHEN IT'S TOO HOT TO COOK

WHAT TO TAKE FOR POT LUCK

LEFTOVER MAKEOVER

COMPANY & HOLIDAY PLANNING

OCCASION: ______________________________ DATE: ______

GUESTS: ______________________________

____

ALLERGIES/SPECIAL DIETS: ______________________________

____

MENU:

OCCASION: ______________________________ DATE: ______

GUESTS: ______________________________

____

ALLERGIES/SPECIAL DIETS: ______________________________

____

MENU:

COMPANY & HOLIDAY PLANNING

OCCASION: ______________________________ DATE: ______

GUESTS: ______________________________

____

ALLERGIES/SPECIAL DIETS: ______________________________

____

MENU:

________	________	________
________	________	________
________	________	________
________	________	________

OCCASION: ______________________________ DATE: ______

GUESTS: ______________________________

____

ALLERGIES/SPECIAL DIETS: ______________________________

____

MENU:

________	________	________
________	________	________
________	________	________
________	________	________

COMPANY & HOLIDAY PLANNING

OCCASION: ____ DATE: ______

GUESTS: ____

____

ALLERGIES/SPECIAL DIETS: ____

____

MENU:

___________________ ___________________ ___________________

___________________ ___________________ ___________________

___________________ ___________________ ___________________

___________________ ___________________ ___________________

OCCASION: ____ DATE: ______

GUESTS: ____

____

ALLERGIES/SPECIAL DIETS: ____

____

MENU:

___________________ ___________________ ___________________

___________________ ___________________ ___________________

___________________ ___________________ ___________________

___________________ ___________________ ___________________

COMPANY & HOLIDAY PLANNING

OCCASION: ______________________________ DATE: ______

GUESTS: ______________________________

____

ALLERGIES/SPECIAL DIETS: ______________________________

____

MENU:

________	________	________
________	________	________
________	________	________
________	________	________

OCCASION: ______________________________ DATE: ______

GUESTS: ______________________________

____

ALLERGIES/SPECIAL DIETS: ______________________________

____

MENU:

________	________	________
________	________	________
________	________	________
________	________	________

COMPANY & HOLIDAY PLANNING

OCCASION: ____ DATE: ______

GUESTS: ____

____

ALLERGIES/SPECIAL DIETS: ____

____

MENU:

____________	____________	____________
____________	____________	____________
____________	____________	____________
____________	____________	____________

OCCASION: ____ DATE: ______

GUESTS: ____

____

ALLERGIES/SPECIAL DIETS: ____

____

MENU:

____________	____________	____________
____________	____________	____________
____________	____________	____________
____________	____________	____________

RECIPE LOCATOR

Recipe Name	Cookbook/Website

FAVORITE RECIPES

Recipe Name: ____

*Serves:*________ *Prep Time*____________ *Cook Time* ______________

Ingredients:

Directions:

Notes:

FAVORITE RECIPES

Recipe Name: ____

*Serves:*_______ *Prep Time*__________ *Cook Time* ____________

Ingredients:

Directions:

Notes:

FAVORITE RECIPES

Recipe Name: ____

*Serves:*_______ *Prep Time*__________ *Cook Time* ____________

Ingredients:

Directions:

Notes:

FAVORITE RECIPES

Recipe Name: ____

*Serves:*________ *Prep Time*____________ *Cook Time* ______________

Ingredients:

Directions:

Notes:

FAVORITE RECIPES

Recipe Name: ____

*Serves:*________ *Prep Time*____________ *Cook Time* ______________

Ingredients:

Directions:

Notes:

NOTES

NOTES

SEASONAL PRODUCE

WHAT TO BUY WHEN

WINTER

- Beets
- Grapefruit
- Kiwi Fruit
- Leeks
- Lemons
- Oranges
- Parsnips
- Pears
- Potatoes
- Brussels Sprouts
- Sweet Potatoes
- Winter Squash
- Pumpkin
- Rutabagas
- Yams

SPRING

- Apricots
- Asparagus
- Broccoli
- Green Beans
- Mangoes
- Mushrooms
- Peas
- Radishes
- Rhubarb
- Spinach
- Strawberries
- Swiss Chard

SUMMER

- Avocados
- Bell Peppers
- Berries
- Cantaloupe
- Cherries
- Corn
- Cucumbers
- Eggplant
- Green Beans
- Honeydew
- Kiwi Fruit
- Okra
- Peaches
- Plums
- Summer Squash
- Tomatoes
- Watermelon

FALL

- Apples
- Beets
- Broccoli
- Cauliflower
- Cranberries
- Grapes
- Kale
- Mushrooms
- Potatoes
- Sweet Potatoes
- Winter Squash
- Parsnips
- Pears
- Pumpkin
- Rutabagas
- Yams
- Turnips

NOTES

SHOPPING LIST

SHOPPING LIST

SHOPPING LIST

SHOPPING LIST

SHOPPING LIST

SHOPPING LIST

SHOPPING LIST

SHOPPING LIST

SHOPPING LIST

SHOPPING LIST

SHOPPING LIST

SHOPPING LIST

SHOPPING LIST

SHOPPING LIST

SHOPPING LIST

SHOPPING LIST

SHOPPING LIST

SHOPPING LIST

SHOPPING LIST

SHOPPING LIST

SHOPPING LIST

SHOPPING LIST

SHOPPING LIST

SHOPPING LIST

SHOPPING LIST

SHOPPING LIST

SHOPPING LIST

SHOPPING LIST

Made in United States
Cleveland, OH
06 November 2026

47789602R00082